THE

ULTIMATE 30-DAY WEIGHT LOSS GUIDE:

TRANSFORM YOUR BODY AND LIFE

ISBN : 9798329430080
First edition ©2024.
Imprint: Independently published

Chief Editor:
Josia pd John
josiajohn735@gmail.com
Dar es salaam - Tanzania
Tel: +255 758588127/ +255 693522834

"The Ultimate 30-Day Weight Loss Guide: Transform Your Body and Life"

Dedication

To all those who have embarked on the challenging journey of transforming their bodies and lives,

This book is dedicated to you—those who dare to dream of a healthier, fitter, and more vibrant version of themselves. It is for those who have taken that first step towards a better future, even when the path seemed steep and uncertain.

Your dedication to self-improvement, your unwavering commitment to change, and your resilience in the face of obstacles are nothing short of inspiring. Your journey is a testament to the incredible strength that resides within each of us, waiting to be awakened.

May this book be your guiding light on this 30-day voyage, offering knowledge, motivation, and practical strategies to help you realize your weight loss goals. But beyond the scales and measurements, may it also inspire you to embrace a healthier, happier, and more fulfilling life.

Remember, the transformation you seek is not just physical—it's a profound shift that encompasses body, mind, and spirit. Your persistence and determination are the keys to unlocking your true potential.

With admiration for your courage and a belief in your limitless potential,

[Prophet PD John]

Preface

Welcome to *"The Ultimate 30-Day Weight Loss Guide: Transform Your Body and Life."* This book is not just about losing weight; it's about embarking on a transformative journey that can redefine your relationship with your body, your health, and your life as a whole.

In a world filled with quick fixes and fad diets, this book takes a different approach. It's rooted in science, practicality, and the understanding that sustainable change takes time. Our goal is to provide you with the knowledge, tools, and motivation to not only shed unwanted pounds in a healthy way but also to adopt a lasting lifestyle that empowers you to thrive.

Before you dive into the chapters that follow, it's essential to grasp the philosophy behind this guide. The journey we're about to embark upon is not a sprint; it's a marathon. It's about making informed choices, cultivating healthy habits, and embracing a mindset that supports your goals.

We'll delve into the science of weight loss, explore the importance of nutrition, exercise, and mindset, and equip you with practical strategies for success. However, remember that there's no one-size-fits-all solution. Your journey is unique, and we encourage you to personalize the advice and techniques to suit your needs and preferences.

Throughout this book, you'll find valuable information, real-life success stories, expert insights, and actionable steps. But remember, knowledge alone is not enough. It's your commitment, determination, and daily actions that will lead to real change.

As you read these pages, keep in mind that this 30-day guide is just the beginning. It's a launchpad for a lifetime of health and well-being. Your transformation doesn't end when these 30 days do; it continues for as long as you choose to prioritize your health.

So, embrace this journey with an open heart and a willingness to change. You have the power to transform not only your body but your entire life. Let's begin this incredible adventure together.

With enthusiasm for your success and well-being,

[Prophet PD John]

Acknowledgments

Creating *"The Ultimate 30-Day Weight Loss Guide: Transform Your Body and Life"* was a labor of love and a collective effort. I would like to express my heartfelt gratitude to everyone who contributed to the realization of this project, directly or indirectly.

First and foremost, I want to thank the readers and those who embark on this transformative journey. Your trust in this guide and your commitment to improving your health and well-being are the driving force behind this book.

I extend my deepest appreciation to the experts and professionals whose knowledge and insights have enriched the content within these pages. Your dedication to the fields of nutrition, fitness, psychology, and health has been instrumental in shaping this comprehensive guide.

A special thank you to the individuals who shared their personal weight loss success stories. Your openness and willingness to inspire others are truly commendable.

I would also like to acknowledge the editorial and publishing team who worked tirelessly to refine and present this information in its best form. Your attention to detail and commitment to quality are evident throughout this book.

To my family and friends, thank you for your unwavering support and encouragement during this creative journey. Your belief in the importance of sharing knowledge and helping others has been a source of motivation.

Lastly, I want to express my gratitude to the countless individuals who have dedicated their lives to researching and promoting health and well-being. Your work has paved the way for a better understanding of the complex interplay between nutrition, exercise, and mental well-being.

As we embark on this transformative path together, I am humbled by the collective effort that has gone into making this guide a reality. It is my hope that it will serve as a valuable resource for those seeking to improve their lives and health.

With sincere appreciation and warm regards,

[Prophet PD John]

Table of Contents

Introduction

I can certainly help you create an outline for a book introduction on ***"The Ultimate 30-Day Weight Loss Guide: Transform your Body and Life."*** However, writing 3000 words here isn't feasible. I can provide you with an outline, and you can use it as a starting point for your introduction:

Introduction: Transforming Your Body and Life in 30 Days

I. The Obesity Epidemic and the Need for Sustainable Weight Loss

In today's world, we are confronted by an obesity epidemic of staggering proportions. While we are undoubtedly living in an age of unprecedented convenience, it has come at a grave cost to our health. The pervasive nature of fast food, sedentary lifestyles, and the constant bombardment of processed, high-calorie foods has led us to a crisis point. Obesity is no longer just a concern; it's a global pandemic.

The Obesity Epidemic: A Looming Crisis

Imagine walking through the bustling streets of a city, where every corner houses a fast-food joint. Tempting aromas waft through the air, and vibrant advertisements display mouthwatering burgers, fries, and sugary beverages. In this landscape, it's all too easy for daily nutrition to take a backseat.

Our modern environment entices us with the promise of instant gratification, and it's no surprise that many have fallen prey to the trappings of convenience. The obesity epidemic is no longer confined to specific age groups, genders, or regions—it's an equal-opportunity health crisis that affects people worldwide.

The Health Implications of Excess Weight

Close your eyes for a moment and picture a backpack. Now, imagine carrying that backpack everywhere you go, 24/7. With each step, it grows heavier, straining your back and affecting your overall well-being. That's what carrying excess weight feels like.

Excess weight isn't merely an issue of aesthetics; it's a profound threat to our health. Obesity is closely linked to a host of debilitating conditions, including heart disease, diabetes, hypertension, and even some types of cancer. Our bodies are not designed to bear this extra burden, and it takes a toll on our physical and mental health.

The Challenge of Sustainable Weight Loss

Consider a mountain climber facing a towering peak. Each step is a struggle, but the view from the top promises incredible rewards. Similarly, embarking on a weight loss journey can feel like a daunting climb. It's challenging, but the transformation that awaits is worth every effort.

Losing weight is a goal many aspire to achieve, yet it's often marred by misconceptions, quick fixes, and unsustainable approaches. Crash diets, extreme exercise regimens, and **"miracle"** supplements promise rapid results, but they often lead to disappointment and health risks. Sustainable weight loss is not a sprint; it's a marathon.

The Role of Diet and Exercise in Weight Management

Think of your body as a finely tuned machine, and the fuel you put into it as the key to its performance. If you pour low-quality fuel into a high-performance car, it won't run optimally. Similarly, the food you consume plays a pivotal role in how your body functions.

Diet and exercise are the cornerstones of weight management. What we eat and how we move profoundly impact our weight, energy levels, and overall well-being. Through this guide, we will explore how to harness the power of nutrition and physical activity to transform your body and life in just 30 days.

As we delve into the science, strategies, and personalized approaches to weight loss, remember that you are not alone on this journey. With the right knowledge, dedication, and support, you can overcome the challenges of the obesity epidemic and achieve sustainable, transformative results in just 30 days. It's time to reclaim your health and vitality.

II. The Science Behind Rapid Weight Loss within 30 Days

In the quest to transform your body and life in just 30 days, it's essential to understand the science that underpins this ambitious goal. While the idea of rapid weight loss might seem daunting, it is indeed achievable when approached with the right knowledge and strategies.

Understanding How Our Bodies Store and Burn Fat

Imagine your body as a finely tuned furnace, continuously converting fuel into energy. At the heart of this process lies fat, a stored form of energy. When we consume more calories than we expend, the excess is stored as fat. Conversely, when we create a calorie deficit, our bodies tap into these fat reserves for energy.

This fundamental concept is at the core of weight loss. By comprehending how your body stores and burns fat, you gain the power to harness this process to your advantage.

The Concept of Caloric Deficit

Creating a caloric deficit—where you consume fewer calories than you burn—is the key to weight loss. It's like repaying that debt, and your body turns to its fat stores to make up the difference. This concept forms the foundation of successful, sustainable weight loss.

Metabolism and its Impact on Weight Loss

Consider your metabolism as the engine that drives your body's energy expenditure. It's the sum of all the processes your body undergoes to maintain life. Your metabolism plays a significant role in determining how quickly or slowly you burn calories.

Metabolism varies from person to person, influenced by factors like age, genetics, and muscle mass. Understanding your metabolism can help tailor your weight loss approach to maximize results.

The 30-Day Timeframe: Benefits and Limitations

Rapid weight loss within 30 days offers both advantages and challenges. On one hand, the short timeframe can provide motivation and a sense of achievement. It can jumpstart your journey and serve as a powerful catalyst for long-term change.

However, it's essential to recognize the limitations. While significant progress is possible, it's unlikely to reach your ultimate weight loss goals in just 30 days. Instead, view this as a crucial step toward a healthier, more sustainable lifestyle.

Balancing Speed and Safety in Weight Loss

Imagine embarking on a road trip—you want to reach your destination efficiently, but you also want to arrive safely. Similarly, in your weight loss journey, speed and safety must be balanced.

Rapid weight loss should prioritize health and well-being. Extreme measures or crash diets can lead to nutrient deficiencies, muscle loss, and other health risks. The goal is not just to lose weight quickly but to do so in a manner that ensures your body's health and vitality.

In the following sections of this guide, we will explore in-depth strategies for creating a caloric deficit, boosting metabolism, and optimizing your 30-day transformation. With the right knowledge and approach, you can achieve rapid, safe, and sustainable weight loss, setting the stage for a healthier and happier life.

III. The Importance of Consulting a Healthcare Professional

Embarking on a 30-day weight loss journey is an admirable goal, but it's essential to recognize that your health is the most valuable asset you possess. To navigate the complexities of this transformation safely and effectively, the guidance of a healthcare professional is invaluable.

The Role of Healthcare Professionals in Weight Management

Imagine setting out on a challenging expedition through uncharted territory. In this journey to transform your body, healthcare professionals serve as experienced guides who know the terrain, the potential hazards, and the safest routes to success.

Healthcare professionals, such as doctors, registered dietitians, and fitness trainers, play a pivotal role in weight management. They possess the knowledge and expertise to assess your unique health needs, guide you toward evidence-based practices, and monitor your progress to ensure your safety.

The Dangers of Crash Dieting and Extreme Exercise

Consider a high-stakes race where the competitors sprint at full speed from the start. While it may seem like a path to victory, it often leads to burnout, injuries, and exhaustion. Similarly, crash dieting and extreme exercise regimens can yield quick results, but they come with significant risks.

Consulting a healthcare professional helps you avoid the pitfalls of extreme approaches. Crash dieting can lead to nutrient deficiencies, muscle loss, and a cycle of yo-yo dieting. Extreme exercise can result in injuries and burnout. Healthcare professionals provide a balanced, sustainable, and safe path to weight loss.

Assessing Individual Health and Fitness Levels

Imagine two individuals, each with distinct medical histories, genetic predispositions, and physical abilities. Their weight loss needs and approaches will inevitably differ. Just as a tailor customizes a suit, healthcare professionals tailor weight loss plans to individual needs.

Before embarking on your 30-day journey, a healthcare professional will assess your current health and fitness levels. They consider factors like medical conditions, medications, allergies, and past dieting experiences to create a personalized plan that maximizes your success while safeguarding your well-being.

Creating a Personalized 30-Day Weight Loss Plan

Think of your weight loss plan as a roadmap to your destination. A one-size-fits-all approach is like using a generic map that doesn't account for the unique features of your journey. A healthcare professional, however, provides a customized roadmap designed to lead you to your goals.

Your personalized 30-day weight loss plan will incorporate dietary recommendations, exercise routines, and strategies to create a sustainable caloric deficit. It takes into account your preferences, limitations, and long-term goals to ensure success.

Monitoring Progress and Making Adjustments

Imagine driving a car with a skilled mechanic in the passenger seat. As you navigate the journey, the mechanic continually assesses the engine's performance and makes real-time adjustments to optimize efficiency. Healthcare professionals serve a similar role in your weight loss journey.

Throughout your 30-day transformation, healthcare professionals will monitor your progress, ensuring that you stay on track and make necessary adjustments to your plan. This ongoing support enhances the likelihood of success and minimizes setbacks.

Safeguarding Your Health During the Transformation

Imagine a safety net beneath a tightrope walker, ready to catch them in case of a misstep. Healthcare professionals provide that safety net during your weight loss journey, ensuring that your health remains the top priority.

As you transform your body in 30 days, your healthcare professional will safeguard your health by addressing any concerns that may arise. They can help prevent complications, manage side effects, and ensure that your journey is not only successful but also safe.

Incorporating the guidance and support of healthcare professionals into your weight loss journey is not a sign of weakness but a testament to your commitment to health and well-being. It's a powerful partnership that enhances your chances of achieving your goals while maintaining your most precious asset—your health.

Part 1:

Preparing for Your 30-Day Weight Loss Journey

Chapter 1:

Assessing Your Current State

A. The Science of Body Composition

Defining Body Composition: Body composition refers to the proportion of fat and non-fat mass in your body. Understanding this composition is essential because it goes beyond just measuring weight on a scale; it provides a more comprehensive view of your health and fitness.

- Difference Between Fat and Lean Mass: Fat mass represents the amount of body fat you carry, while lean mass includes everything else in your body, such as muscles, bones, organs, and water. The balance between these two components is vital for overall health and well-being.

- Genetic Influence on Body Composition: Genetics can play a significant role in determining your body composition. Some people may naturally have a higher propensity to store fat, while others may have a genetic advantage when it comes to building lean muscle. Recognizing these genetic factors helps you better understand your starting point in your weight loss journey.

This section of Chapter 1 sets the stage for readers to appreciate the importance of assessing their body composition as a foundational step in their 30-day weight loss journey. It explains the basic concepts and factors that influence body composition, encouraging readers to consider their unique starting point before setting goals and embarking on their transformation.

B. Methods for Measuring Body Composition

- **Discussing Common Methods:** This section explores various methods used to assess body composition. It provides an overview of the following common techniques:

1. Body Mass Index (BMI): BMI is a simple formula that compares your weight to your height. It's widely used but has limitations, as it doesn't distinguish between fat and muscle.

2. Skinfold Measurements: Skinfold measurements involve using calipers to measure the thickness of skinfolds at specific sites on the body. These measurements can estimate body fat percentage.

3. Bioelectrical Impedance: Bioelectrical impedance devices measure the resistance of electrical flow through your body. They estimate body fat based on the principle that fat conducts less electricity than lean tissue.

4. Dual-Energy X-ray Absorptiometry (DEXA): DEXA scans are highly accurate and provide detailed information about your body composition, including bone density, fat, and lean mass.

- Pros and Cons: For each measurement method, this section discusses the advantages and drawbacks. For example, BMI is easy to calculate but lacks precision, while DEXA is highly accurate but requires specialized equipment.

- Emphasizing Accuracy: This section underscores the importance of choosing a measurement method that aligns with your goals and emphasizes the significance of accuracy. A precise assessment of body composition allows for better tracking of progress and helps in tailoring your weight loss plan to your specific needs.

This part of Chapter 1 equips readers with knowledge about the various methods available to measure body composition. By understanding the pros and cons of each method, readers can make informed decisions about which approach best suits their needs and objectives in their 30-day weight loss journey.

C. Interpreting Your Body Composition Data

- **Analyzing Results:** After undergoing body composition assessments, this section guides readers on how to interpret the data they receive. It emphasizes the importance of understanding what the numbers mean in the context of their health and fitness goals.

- **Identifying Areas for Improvement:** Readers are encouraged to identify specific areas where they may need improvement based on their body composition results. For instance, they might recognize a high body fat percentage or a deficit in lean muscle mass.

- **Understanding Health and Fitness Implications:** This section delves into how body composition directly impacts overall health and fitness. It explains that having an excess of body fat, especially around vital organs, can increase the risk of various health conditions. On the other hand, having a healthy ratio of lean muscle can enhance metabolism and overall well-being.

By helping readers analyze their body composition data, identify areas for improvement, and grasp the implications for their health and fitness, this section prepares them to set informed and realistic goals for their 30-day weight loss journey. It underscores the connection between body composition and well-being, motivating readers to take action towards positive change.

III. Setting Realistic Weight Loss Goals

A. The Power of Goal Setting

- The Psychological Impact of Goals: This part explores how setting and achieving goals can have a profound psychological impact. It highlights how having clear objectives can provide motivation, focus, and a sense of accomplishment throughout the weight loss journey.

- Importance of Realistic Goals: Readers are introduced to the idea that setting realistic goals is not only more attainable but also sustainable. Unrealistic goals can lead to frustration and disappointment, while realistic goals provide a clear path to success.

B. Assessing Your Personal Goals

- Identifying Motivations: This section encourages readers to reflect on their personal motivations for weight loss. Whether it's improving health, enhancing appearance, or boosting fitness levels, understanding these motivations serves as a strong foundation for goal setting.

- SMART Criteria: Readers are introduced to the SMART criteria (Specific, Measurable, Achievable, Relevant, Time-bound) as a framework for defining their goals. This approach helps ensure that goals are well-defined, trackable, and realistic.

C. Understanding Healthy Weight Loss Rates

- **Explaining Recommended Rates:** This part provides insight into what constitutes a healthy rate of weight loss. It emphasizes the importance of gradual and sustainable weight loss over rapid, extreme methods.

- **Factors Affecting Rate:** Readers learn that the rate of weight loss can vary from person to person. Factors like starting weight, metabolism, and individual circumstances can influence how quickly or slowly one can expect to shed pounds.

By guiding readers through the process of setting realistic weight loss goals, this section empowers them to define their objectives clearly, align them with their motivations, and understand the importance of pursuing healthy, sustainable changes during their 30-day weight loss journey.

D. Creating Short-term and Long-term Goals

- The Importance of Milestones: This part underscores the value of breaking down your weight loss journey into manageable milestones. It explains that setting milestones helps you maintain focus, provides a sense of achievement along the way, and keeps you motivated.

- Setting Short-term Goals: Readers are encouraged to define specific, achievable goals for their 30-day weight loss journey. These short-term goals serve as building blocks towards broader success.

- Long-term Goals for Ongoing Success: Beyond the 30-day period, this section highlights the importance of setting long-term goals to sustain your progress. It emphasizes that long-term goals help you maintain healthy habits and continue your journey toward a healthier lifestyle.

IV. Tracking Progress and Adjusting Goals

A. The Role of Progress Tracking

- Continuous Monitoring: This part explains why ongoing monitoring of your weight loss journey is crucial. Regular tracking allows you to observe your progress, identify trends, and make data-driven decisions.

- Tools and Methods: Readers are introduced to various tools and methods for tracking progress, such as keeping journals, using fitness apps, or taking progress photos. These techniques enable you to visualize your journey and stay accountable.

B. Celebrating Achievements

- **Recognizing Small Victories:** Celebrating small achievements along the way is essential for motivation. This section explains how acknowledging even minor successes can boost your confidence and keep you inspired.

- **Positive Reinforcement:** Positive reinforcement, in the form of rewards or self-praise, is highlighted as a powerful tool for sustaining motivation. It keeps you engaged and dedicated to your goals.

C. Adaptation and Flexibility

- **Need for Goal Adjustment:** This section stresses that circumstances can change during a weight loss journey, such as encountering plateaus or dealing with unexpected life events. It emphasizes that adjusting goals when necessary is a sign of adaptability, not failure.

- **Strategies for Challenges:** Readers are provided with strategies for staying on course during challenging times. These include seeking support from peers or professionals, modifying your approach, and maintaining a growth mindset.

These sections equip readers with the knowledge and tools needed to set, track, and adapt their goals effectively throughout their 30-day weight loss journey. By emphasizing the importance of milestones, progress tracking, and adaptability, readers are well-prepared to overcome obstacles and stay committed to their goals.

V. Summary of Chapter 1

In Chapter 1, we embarked on the crucial first steps of your 30-day weight loss journey, laying the foundation for your success. Here's a recap of the key takeaways from this chapter:

- We emphasized the *importance of self-assessment* as a fundamental aspect of achieving successful weight loss. By understanding where you currently stand in terms of your body composition and personal goals, you are better equipped to move forward effectively.

- We explored the intricacies of *body composition,* delving into the science of fat mass and lean mass. Understanding your body's unique composition is essential for making informed decisions about your weight loss journey.

- You were introduced to various *methods for measuring body composition,* such as BMI, skinfold measurements, bioelectrical impedance, and DEXA scans. Each method has its pros and cons, and choosing the right one for your needs is essential.

- After assessing your body composition, we moved on to *setting realistic weight loss goals.* We highlighted the powerful psychological impact of goal setting and stressed the importance of setting objectives that are specific, measurable, achievable, relevant, and time-bound (SMART).

- We discussed the *rate of healthy weight loss* and explained why gradual, sustainable progress is preferable to rapid, extreme approaches. Factors affecting the rate of weight loss, including your starting weight and metabolism, were also explored.

- You learned the significance of creating both *short-term and long-term goals* to keep you motivated and focused throughout your journey. Short-term goals help you track your progress, while long-term goals ensure that you sustain your achievements over time.

- The importance of *tracking progress and adjusting goals* as your journey unfolds was emphasized. Continuous monitoring, celebrating achievements, and adapting to challenges are all critical components of a successful weight loss plan.

In conclusion, Chapter 1 has set the stage for your 30-day weight loss journey by providing you with the knowledge and tools to assess your current state, define realistic goals, and understand the significance of body composition. Armed with this foundation, you are ready to move forward with confidence and purpose, knowing that success is within reach.

Chapter 2:

Creating Your Weight Loss Plan

I. Introduction to Chapter 2

In the previous chapter, you laid the groundwork for your 30-day weight loss journey by understanding your body composition and setting realistic goals. Now, in Chapter 2, we embark on the exciting phase of crafting your personalized weight loss plan. This chapter is pivotal in your transformation as it forms the blueprint for your success.

We will explore the critical elements that make up a well-structured weight loss plan and guide you in tailoring it to your unique needs and preferences. Your personalized plan will encompass not only dietary choices and exercise routines but also the psychological aspects of motivation.

Join us as we delve into the significance of a thoughtfully crafted weight loss plan and how it serves as your compass on this transformative journey. By the end of this chapter, you will be equipped with a comprehensive plan that is not only effective but also sustainable, setting you firmly on the path to achieving your goals in the next 30 days and beyond.

II. The Role of Calorie Deficit and Macronutrients

A. Understanding Calorie Deficit

- **Defining a Calorie Deficit:** A calorie deficit occurs when you consume fewer calories than your body needs to maintain its current weight. In essence, you're creating an energy shortfall that forces your body to tap into its stored fat for fuel.

Example: Imagine your daily energy expenditure is 2,000 calories, but you consume only 1,800 calories in a day. This 200-calorie deficit, if sustained over time, leads to weight loss.

- The Fat Loss Mechanism: When you maintain a calorie deficit, your body turns to its fat stores to make up for the energy shortfall. It breaks down fat into usable energy, which leads to fat loss.

Example: Think of your body fat as a backup fuel tank. When you create a calorie deficit, your body starts drawing from this reserve to meet its energy needs, resulting in reduced body fat over time.

- Balancing Calorie Intake and Expenditure: Achieving a calorie deficit involves finding the right balance between the calories you consume through food and beverages and the calories you burn through daily activities and exercise.

B. The Essentials of Macronutrients

- **Explaining Macronutrients:** Macronutrients are the three primary components of the foods you eat: carbohydrates, proteins, and fats. Each macronutrient plays a unique role in the body's functions.

- **Carbohydrates** provide energy for daily activities and exercise.

- **Proteins** are essential for building and repairing tissues, including muscles.

- **Fats** are a concentrated source of energy and are crucial for various bodily functions, such as hormone production and nutrient absorption.

- **Determining Ideal Macronutrient Ratios:** Your ideal macronutrient ratios can vary depending on your goals and preferences. For weight loss, some people may benefit from a balanced approach, while others might opt for a higher protein intake to support muscle preservation.

Example: If you're engaging in regular strength training during your 30-day weight loss journey, you might choose a diet with a higher protein content to help maintain muscle mass.

C. Portion Control and Mindful Eating

- **Impact of Portion Sizes:** The size of your food portions directly affects your calorie intake. Larger portions often lead to overconsumption of calories, making it challenging to maintain a calorie deficit.

  Example: A large serving of pasta might contain significantly more calories than a smaller portion of the same dish.

- **Mindful Eating Techniques:** Practicing mindful eating involves paying full attention to the eating experience. Techniques include savoring each bite, eating slowly, and being mindful of hunger and fullness cues.

  Example: When practicing mindful eating, you might notice that you feel satisfied with a smaller portion of a favorite dessert, preventing overindulgence.

- Controlling Portions When Dining Out: Dining out can present challenges in portion control. Tips for controlling portions include sharing dishes with others, ordering appetizers or smaller portions, and asking for a to-go container to save half of your meal for later.

Example: When dining out at a restaurant known for generous portions, you might split an entrée with a friend to avoid overeating.

This section provides readers with a fundamental understanding of how a calorie deficit and macronutrients influence weight loss. It also offers practical advice on portion control and mindful eating to help readers make informed dietary choices during their 30-day weight loss journey.

III. Personalizing Your Diet and Exercise Plan

A. Crafting Your Diet Plan

- Aligning Diet with Goals and Preferences: Your diet plan should be a reflection of your specific goals and personal preferences. Whether you're aiming for weight loss, muscle gain, or improved overall health, tailoring your diet to your objectives ensures that it's both effective and sustainable.

Example: If your goal is weight loss and you prefer a vegetarian diet, crafting a meal plan rich in plant-based foods that aligns with your calorie deficit target can be a sustainable approach.

- Selecting Nutrient-Dense Foods: Nutrient-dense foods are those that provide essential nutrients (vitamins, minerals, fiber) with relatively few calories. Incorporating these foods into your diet helps support weight loss while ensuring you receive necessary nutrients.

Example: Opting for a colorful salad with a variety of vegetables, lean protein, and a light dressing can be a nutrient-dense choice compared to a calorie-dense fast-food meal.

- Creating a Balanced Meal Plan: Balance is key in a sustainable diet plan. This involves including a variety of food groups to meet your nutritional needs. A balanced meal plan considers your daily calorie target, macronutrient ratios, and portion sizes.

Example: Balancing a meal by including lean protein (chicken breast), carbohydrates (quinoa), and healthy fats (avocado) provides a well-rounded and satisfying plate.

B. Tailoring Your Exercise Routine

- Assessing Fitness Level and Appropriate Exercises: To ensure a safe and effective workout routine, it's essential to assess your current fitness level. This evaluation helps you choose exercises that match your capabilities and gradually progress to more challenging workouts.

Example: If you're new to exercise, starting with low-impact activities like brisk walking or swimming can prevent injury and build a foundation for more intense workouts.

- Incorporating Cardiovascular and Strength Training: A well-rounded exercise plan includes both cardiovascular and strength training exercises. Cardio workouts improve endurance and burn calories, while strength training builds lean muscle mass and boosts metabolism.

Example: Your 30-day plan might include a mix of activities like jogging or cycling (cardio) and bodyweight exercises or weightlifting (strength training) to achieve a balanced approach.

- Setting Realistic Workout Goals: It's crucial to establish clear, achievable workout goals for the

30-day period. Realistic goals keep you motivated and provide a sense of accomplishment as you progress.

Example: A realistic goal might be to increase the number of push-ups you can do from 10 to 20 within the 30-day period.

C. The Role of Rest and Recovery

- Significance of Rest and Sleep: Rest days and adequate sleep are often underestimated aspects of a successful weight loss plan. Rest allows your muscles to recover, reducing the risk of injury, and sleep is essential for hormonal balance and overall well-being.

Example: Prioritizing 7-9 hours of quality sleep per night and incorporating rest days between intense workouts can optimize your recovery.

- Strategies for Promoting Sleep and Recovery: This section offers practical strategies to promote better sleep and recovery, such as establishing a consistent sleep schedule, creating a relaxing bedtime routine, and managing stress.

Example: You might develop a calming bedtime routine that includes reading, gentle stretching, and avoiding screen time to improve your sleep quality.

- Avoiding Overtraining and Burnout: Overtraining can lead to exhaustion, injuries, and burnout. This part discusses the importance of listening to your body's signals and adjusting your exercise routine when needed to prevent overtraining.

Example: If you experience persistent fatigue or muscle soreness, you might reduce workout intensity or schedule additional rest days to avoid overtraining.

This section of Chapter 2 guides readers in creating a personalized diet and exercise plan that aligns with their goals, preferences, and fitness level. By emphasizing balance, realistic goals, and the importance of rest and recovery, it ensures that the plan is both effective and sustainable for their 30-day weight loss journey.

IV. The Psychology of Motivation

A. Understanding Motivation Factors

- **Identifying Motivation Factors:** This section encourages readers to explore and recognize both internal and external factors that drive their motivation. Internal factors might include a desire for improved health, increased self-confidence, or personal fulfillment. External factors could involve support from friends, family, or the desire to participate in a specific event.

Example: An internal motivation factor could be the desire to feel more energetic and confident, while an external factor might be having a workout buddy who keeps you accountable.

- Using Motivations as Tools for Success: Readers learn how to harness their motivations as powerful tools for success. By understanding what truly drives them, they can leverage these motivations to fuel their commitment to their weight loss journey.

Example: If the desire for improved health is a strong internal motivator, it can be used as a daily reminder to make healthier food choices and prioritize regular exercise.

B. Goal Visualization and Affirmations

- Techniques for Goal Visualization: Visualization involves mentally imagining achieving your weight loss goals. This section introduces readers to visualization techniques that help them vividly picture their desired outcomes.

Example: Close your eyes and imagine yourself fitting into those jeans you've always wanted to wear. Visualize the sense of accomplishment and confidence that comes with achieving your goal.

- The Power of Positive Affirmations: Positive affirmations are statements that reinforce your motivation and self-belief. They can boost confidence and remind you of your potential for success.

Example: Repeating affirmations like "I am capable of achieving my goals" or "I am becoming healthier every day" can foster a positive mindset.

- Integration into Daily Routine: Readers are encouraged to integrate goal visualization and affirmations into their daily routines. This practice helps keep their motivation front and center.

C. Overcoming Obstacles and Staying Committed

- **Common Obstacles:** This section addresses common obstacles that individuals encounter during their weight loss journey. Examples include cravings, time constraints, and setbacks. Readers gain insights into strategies for overcoming these challenges.

Example: If cravings for unhealthy snacks are a challenge, you might learn about healthier alternatives and how to manage cravings effectively.

- **Importance of Resilience and Perseverance:** Weight loss journeys are rarely linear. This part emphasizes the importance of resilience and perseverance in the face of setbacks. It's normal to experience plateaus or temporary setbacks, but it's crucial to keep moving forward.

Example: Rather than giving up after a plateau, you might explore adjustments to your diet or exercise routine to break through.

- Building a Support System: Having a support system can be a game-changer. Whether it's friends, family, or a weight loss group, having people who share your goals and provide accountability can significantly enhance your commitment.

Example: Joining a weekly workout class with friends not only provides companionship but also creates a sense of responsibility to attend regularly.

This section of Chapter 2 delves into the psychological aspects of motivation, offering practical guidance on how to identify and utilize motivation factors effectively. It also provides readers with tools like goal visualization, affirmations, and strategies to overcome obstacles, ensuring they stay committed and motivated throughout their 30-day weight loss journey.

V. Summary of Chapter 2

In Chapter 2, we embarked on the essential phase of crafting your personalized weight loss plan, setting the stage for your transformative 30-day journey. Let's recap the key takeaways from this chapter:

- **Calorie Deficit and Macronutrients:** We explored the pivotal role of a calorie deficit in driving fat loss, as well as the significance of understanding macronutrients (carbohydrates, proteins, fats) in creating a balanced diet. By balancing calorie intake and expenditure and selecting nutrient-dense foods, you are equipped with the knowledge to make informed dietary choices.

- **Personalization:** Your weight loss plan is not one-size-fits-all. We highlighted the importance of aligning your diet and exercise plan with your unique goals, preferences, and fitness level. Personalization ensures that your plan is both effective and sustainable.

- **Motivation:** The psychology of motivation was discussed in depth. You learned to identify the internal and external factors that drive your motivation and how to harness these motivations as powerful tools for success. Techniques like goal visualization and positive affirmations were introduced to reinforce your commitment.

- Overcoming Obstacles: Common obstacles in a weight loss journey were addressed, along with strategies for overcoming them. We emphasized the importance of resilience and perseverance in the face of setbacks and the value of building a support system to stay accountable.

As you move forward in your 30-day weight loss journey, remember that the combination of a calorie deficit, a well-balanced diet, personalization, and unwavering motivation forms the foundation of your success. By integrating these principles into your daily routine, you are well-prepared to achieve your goals and transform your life for the better. Stay committed, stay motivated, and keep your eyes on the prize!

Chapter 3:

The Science of Weight Loss

Introduction

Weight loss is a subject of enduring fascination and concern for many individuals. From fad diets and exercise regimens to miracle supplements and cutting-edge surgeries, there's a myriad of approaches to shedding excess pounds. Yet, understanding the fundamental science behind weight loss is paramount for achieving lasting results and maintaining a healthy lifestyle. This chapter delves into three crucial aspects:

1. Metabolism and its Impact on Weight Loss

2. Hormones and Their Role in Weight Regulation

3. Common Misconceptions About Dieting

By exploring these topics in-depth, we can demystify the complexities of weight loss and empower individuals to make informed decisions on their journey towards better health.

Section 1: Metabolism and its Impact on Weight Loss

1.1 What is Metabolism?

Metabolism is the set of biochemical processes that occur within an organism to maintain life. In simpler terms, it's the body's engine responsible for converting food into energy. This energy powers every bodily function, from breathing and digesting food to exercising and thinking. Metabolism can be broadly categorized into two components:

1.1.1 Basal Metabolic Rate (BMR)

Basal Metabolic Rate (BMR) refers to the number of calories your body requires to maintain basic functions while at rest. This includes functions like maintaining body temperature, circulating blood, and repairing cells. BMR accounts for the majority of calories burned daily, approximately 60-75% for most people. Factors influencing BMR include:

- Age: BMR generally decreases with age.

- Gender: Men often have a higher BMR than women due to higher muscle mass.

- Body Composition: Muscle burns more calories at rest than fat, so individuals with more muscle mass have a higher BMR.

- Genetics: Genetic factors can impact your metabolic rate to some extent.

1.1.2 Thermic Effect of Food (TEF)

TEF refers to the energy expended during the digestion and absorption of food. When you eat, your body needs energy to break down and process the nutrients in the food. This accounts for about 10% of your daily calorie expenditure.

1.1.3 Physical Activity

Physical activity, including exercise and daily movements, can significantly influence your metabolism. Activities like jogging, weightlifting, or even fidgeting burn calories and contribute to your overall daily energy expenditure. This component of metabolism is the most variable and controllable, accounting for 15-30% of daily calorie burn.

1.2 Metabolism and Weight Loss

Understanding metabolism is crucial in the context of weight loss because it dictates how many calories your body burns. If you consume more calories than your metabolism burns, the excess is stored as fat, leading to weight gain. Conversely, if you consume fewer calories than your metabolism burns, your body taps into fat stores for energy, resulting in weight loss.

1.2.1 Strategies to Boost Metabolism

- **Regular Exercise:** Engaging in physical activity, especially resistance training, can increase muscle mass and, consequently, BMR.

- **Balanced Diet:** Eating nutrient-dense foods and avoiding crash diets helps maintain metabolic health.

- **Adequate Sleep:** Poor sleep patterns can disrupt hormone regulation and negatively impact metabolism.

- **Hydration:** Staying well-hydrated is essential for efficient metabolic processes.

- **Stress Management:** Chronic stress can elevate cortisol levels, which may lead to weight gain. Stress-reduction techniques like meditation and yoga can help.

Section 2: Hormones and Their Role in Weight Regulation

2.1 Hormones and Weight

Hormones are chemical messengers that regulate various physiological processes in the body. When it comes to weight regulation, several hormones play pivotal roles:

2.1.1 Insulin

Insulin is a hormone produced by the pancreas in response to increased blood sugar levels after eating. Its primary role is to facilitate the uptake of glucose into cells for energy or storage. High insulin levels, often associated with excessive consumption of refined carbohydrates and sugars, can promote fat storage and hinder weight loss.

2.1.2 Leptin

Leptin, often referred to as the "satiety hormone," is produced by fat cells and signals to the brain that you're full. In individuals with obesity, there can be resistance to leptin's effects, leading to overeating and weight gain. Strategies to support healthy leptin function include maintaining a balanced diet and regular exercise.

2.1.3 Ghrelin

Ghrelin is known as the "hunger hormone" because it stimulates appetite. Its levels typically rise before meals and fall after eating. Disruptions in ghrelin regulation can lead to increased appetite and weight gain.

2.1.4 Cortisol

Cortisol is a stress hormone produced by the adrenal glands. Chronic stress can lead to elevated cortisol levels, which may promote fat storage, particularly around the abdominal area. Managing stress through relaxation techniques and adequate sleep is crucial for weight management.

2.2 Hormonal Imbalances and Weight

Hormonal imbalances can significantly impact weight regulation. Conditions like polycystic ovary syndrome (PCOS), thyroid disorders, and insulin resistance can lead to weight gain or hinder weight loss efforts. Addressing these underlying hormonal issues often requires medical intervention and personalized treatment plans.

Section 3: Common Misconceptions About Dieting

3.1 Crash Diets

Misconception: Crash diets promising rapid weight loss are effective long-term solutions.

Reality: Crash diets are typically unsustainable and can lead to muscle loss, nutritional deficiencies, and rebound weight gain. Sustainable weight loss is best achieved through gradual, balanced changes to your diet and lifestyle.

3.2 Starvation Mode

Misconception: Eating too little puts your body into *"starvation mode,"* causing it to conserve fat.

Reality: While prolonged severe calorie restriction can slow metabolism, the concept of ***"starvation mode"*** is often misunderstood. Consistently undereating can hinder weight loss and harm your health.

3.3 Spot Reduction

Misconception: Targeted exercises can burn fat in specific areas of the body.

Reality: Fat loss occurs uniformly across the body, not in specific areas targeted by exercises. Building muscle in specific areas can improve their appearance but won't necessarily burn fat in those regions.

3.4 All Calories are Equal

Misconception: All calories are the same, regardless of their source.

Reality: The quality of calories matters. Nutrient-dense foods provide essential vitamins and minerals that support overall health. A balanced diet with a variety of foods is more effective for long-term health and weight management.

3.5 Supplements and Detoxes

Misconception: Weight loss supplements and detox programs are effective and safe.

Reality: Many supplements and detox programs lack scientific support and can be harmful. A balanced diet and regular exercise are the most effective and sustainable approaches to weight management.

Conclusion

Understanding the science of weight loss is essential for making informed choices on your journey towards a healthier lifestyle. Metabolism, hormones, and common miscon

Chapter 4:

Building a Support System

Introduction

Embarking on a weight loss journey can be challenging, but it becomes significantly more manageable when you have a robust support system in place. Chapter 4 explores the importance of building a support system and offers strategies to do so effectively. Three key aspects of this chapter are:

1. Enlisting Friends and Family for Support

2. Finding a Workout Buddy

3. Joining Weight Loss Communities

Section 1: Enlisting Friends and Family for Support

1.1 The Power of Social Support

Weight loss isn't a solo endeavor. Friends and family can provide invaluable emotional support, motivation, and accountability throughout your journey. Here's how to enlist their support effectively:

1.1.1 Communication

Open and honest communication is key. Share your goals, challenges, and the role you'd like them to play in your weight loss journey. Explain how their support can make a significant difference.

1.1.2 Meal Planning

Involve your loved ones in meal planning and preparation. This fosters a shared commitment to healthier eating habits. Family meals can become opportunities to enjoy nutritious food together.

1.1.3 Active Participation

Encourage your friends and family to participate in physical activities with you. Whether it's going for a walk, hiking, or trying a new sport, involving them in your workouts can make exercise more enjoyable.

1.1.4 Emotional Support

Lean on your support system during challenging times. They can provide encouragement, motivation, and a listening ear when you need it most.

1.2 Overcoming Challenges

While support from friends and family can be invaluable, there may also be challenges, such as:

1.2.1 Unsolicited Advice

Be prepared for well-meaning but unsolicited advice. Politely assert your goals and strategies while appreciating their concern.

1.2.2 Sabotage

Occasionally, loved ones may unknowingly undermine your efforts. Share your boundaries and request their understanding and cooperation.

Section 2: Finding a Workout Buddy

2.1 The Benefits of a Workout Buddy

Having a workout buddy can boost your motivation, accountability, and enjoyment of physical activity. Here's how to find and maintain a workout partnership:

2.1.1 Shared Goals

Find someone with similar fitness goals. Having a common objective creates a sense of camaraderie and mutual support.

2.1.2 Compatibility

Choose a workout buddy whose schedule and exercise preferences align with yours. This ensures consistency in your workouts.

2.1.3 Accountability

Regularly communicate and set workout schedules together. Knowing someone is counting on you can be a powerful motivator to stay committed.

2.1.4 Variety

Exploring different types of physical activity together can keep workouts exciting and prevent boredom.

2.2 Maintaining a Workout Partnership

To ensure a successful workout partnership, consider the following:

2.2.1 Communication

Keep communication channels open. Discuss any changes in schedules, preferences, or goals to avoid misunderstandings.

2.2.2 Flexibility

Be adaptable and understanding. Life can be unpredictable, and occasionally, your workout buddy may need to reschedule.

2.2.3 Encouragement

Support each other's progress and celebrate achievements, no matter how small. Positive reinforcement can strengthen your partnership.

Section 3: Joining Weight Loss Communities

3.1 The Role of Communities

Weight loss communities, whether in-person or online, offer a sense of belonging and shared experience. Here's how to make the most of these communities:

3.1.1 Online Forums and Social Media

Participate in online forums, Facebook groups, or fitness apps dedicated to weight loss. These platforms provide a space for sharing tips, progress, and setbacks.

3.1.2 Local Support Groups

Look for local weight loss or fitness groups that meet in person. These can offer real-world connections and additional accountability.

3.1.3 Accountability Partners

Within these communities, consider finding an accountability partner with similar goals. Regular check-ins and shared progress can be motivating.

3.2 Avoiding Pitfalls

While weight loss communities can be immensely beneficial, it's essential to navigate them mindfully:

3.2.1 Information Overload

Be cautious of information overload. While communities provide valuable insights, not all advice may be suitable for your unique circumstances.

3.2.2 Comparison

Avoid constant comparison to others in the community. Remember that everyone's weight loss journey is individual, and progress may differ.

3.2.3 Negativity

If a community becomes overly negative or competitive, consider seeking a more supportive and constructive environment.

Conclusion

Building a support system is a fundamental component of a successful weight loss journey. Friends, family, workout buddies, and weight loss communities can provide motivation, accountability, and a sense of belonging. By effectively leveraging these sources of support, you can navigate the challenges of weight loss with confidence and perseverance..

Chapter 5:

Preparing Your Kitchen and Pantry

Introduction

One of the most influential factors in your weight loss journey is the environment in which you prepare and consume your meals. Chapter 5 focuses on the importance of setting up a kitchen and pantry that support your health and weight loss goals. The three key aspects explored in this chapter are:

1. **Stocking Up on Healthy Foods**

2. **Eliminating Temptations**

3. **Kitchen Tools and Gadgets for Success**

1.1 The Foundation of Healthy Eating

A well-stocked kitchen and pantry provide the foundation for healthy eating. Here's how to ensure you have the right ingredients at your fingertips:

1.1.1 Fresh Produce

Load up on fresh fruits and vegetables. These should be the cornerstone of your diet, providing essential vitamins, minerals, and fiber.

1.1.2 Lean Protein

Include sources of lean protein like chicken, turkey, fish, beans, and tofu. Protein helps you feel full and supports muscle maintenance.

1.1.3 Whole Grains

Opt for whole grains such as brown rice, quinoa, and whole wheat pasta. They are higher in fiber and nutrients compared to refined grains.

1.1.4 Healthy Fats

Stock up on sources of healthy fats like avocados, nuts, seeds, and olive oil. These fats are essential for overall health.

1.1.5 Low-Calorie Snacks

Have healthy snacks readily available, such as Greek yogurt, hummus, and fresh fruit, to curb cravings between meals.

1.2 Meal Planning

Effective meal planning can simplify healthy eating and reduce the temptation to order takeout or indulge in unhealthy options. Consider the following meal planning strategies:

1.2.1 Weekly Meal Plans

Plan your meals for the week ahead, including breakfast, lunch, dinner, and snacks. This reduces the need for last-minute, less healthy choices.

1.2.2 Portion Control

Pre-portion snacks and meals to avoid overeating. Invest in containers and storage solutions that make portion control easy.

1.2.3 Batch Cooking

Prepare large batches of healthy meals and freeze portions for later. This saves time and prevents you from reaching for less nutritious options when you're busy.

Section 2: Eliminating Temptations

2.1 Out of Sight, Out of Mind

Minimizing the presence of unhealthy foods in your kitchen can reduce temptation. Consider these strategies:

2.1.1 Decluttering

Regularly go through your pantry and refrigerator to remove foods that don't align with your health goals.

2.1.2 Hidden Treasures

If certain unhealthy foods are irresistible to you, keep them out of sight or in less accessible places.

2.1.3 Supportive Household

Discuss your goals with family members or housemates and request their cooperation in not bringing unhealthy foods into the home.

2.2 Mindful Shopping

Practices you implement while shopping can impact your food choices at home:

2.2.1 Shopping List

Always shop with a list and stick to it. This reduces impulse purchases of unhealthy items.

2.2.2 Perimeter Shopping

Most grocery stores place fresh produce, lean proteins, and dairy along the perimeter. Spend the majority of your time shopping in these areas.

Section 3: Kitchen Tools and Gadgets for Success

3.1 Equipping Your Kitchen

Investing in the right kitchen tools and gadgets can make healthy cooking more convenient and enjoyable:

3.1.1 Food Scale

A food scale helps with portion control, ensuring you don't overeat.

3.1.2 Blender

A blender is excellent for making smoothies, soups, and healthy sauces.

3.1.3 Steamer

A steamer makes cooking vegetables easy while preserving their nutrients.

3.1.4 Non-Stick Cookware

Non-stick pans reduce the need for excess cooking oils and fats.

3.2 Meal Prep Tools

Consider these tools to streamline meal prep:

3.2.1 Meal Prep Containers

Invest in high-quality meal prep containers that are microwave and dishwasher safe for storing pre-made meals.

3.2.2 Slow Cooker

A slow cooker allows for easy, hands-off cooking of nutritious meals.

3.2.3 Spiralizer

A spiralizer can turn vegetables into healthy, low-carb substitutes for pasta.

Conclusion

A well-prepared kitchen and pantry can significantly contribute to your success in achieving and maintaining a healthy weight. Stocking up on nutritious foods, eliminating temptations, and equipping your kitchen with the right tools are essential steps in creating an environment that supports your health and weight loss goals. By taking control of your kitchen, you take a significant step towards taking control of your health.

Part 2:

Nutrition for Rapid
Weight Loss

Chapter 6:

Understanding Calories

Introduction

In your quest for rapid weight loss, understanding the role of calories is paramount. Chapter 6 delves into the science of calories and how to calculate your daily calorie needs. This knowledge will serve as the foundation for making informed dietary choices and achieving your weight loss goals.

Section 1: The Science of Calories

1.1 What is a Calorie?

A calorie is a unit of measurement for energy. In the context of nutrition, it refers to the energy derived from the foods and beverages we consume. Understanding calories is crucial because weight loss fundamentally boils down to managing your calorie balance.

1.2 The Caloric Value of Macronutrients

Different macronutrients provide varying amounts of energy per gram:

- **Carbohydrates:** Approximately 4 calories per gram.

- **Proteins:** Approximately 4 calories per gram.

- **Fats:** Approximately 9 calories per gram.

- **Alcohol:** Approximately 7 calories per gram.

This differentiation in calorie content underscores the importance of a balanced diet.

1.3 Calorie Expenditure

Calorie expenditure refers to the number of calories your body burns in a day. This expenditure is composed of three primary components:

1.3.1 Basal Metabolic Rate (BMR)

BMR is the number of calories your body needs to maintain basic functions at rest, such as breathing and cell maintenance.

1.3.2 Physical Activity

Physical activity encompasses all the calories burned through exercise, daily movements, and workouts.

1.3.3 Thermic Effect of Food (TEF)

TEF accounts for the calories expended during digestion and absorption of the foods you eat.

Section 2: Calculating Your Daily Calorie Needs

2.1 Determining Your Basal Metabolic Rate (BMR)

Calculating your BMR provides a baseline for understanding your calorie needs. There are various formulas to estimate BMR, with the Harris-Benedict equation being one of the most commonly used. It takes into account your age, gender, weight, and height.

2.1.1 Harris-Benedict Equation for BMR

For men: BMR = 88.362 + (13.397 x weight in kg) + (4.799 x height in cm) - (5.677 x age in years)

For women: BMR = 447.593 + (9.247 x weight in kg) + (3.098 x height in cm) - (4.330 x age in years)

2.2 Accounting for Physical Activity

Once you have your BMR, you'll need to factor in your physical activity level to determine your total daily calorie needs. Common activity levels include:

- Sedentary (little to no exercise)

- Lightly active (light exercise or sports 1-3 days a week)

- Moderately active (moderate exercise or sports 3-5 days a week)

- Very active (hard exercise or sports 6-7 days a week)

- Super active (very hard exercise, physical job, or training twice a day)

You can multiply your BMR by an activity factor that corresponds to your activity level to get your daily calorie needs.

2.3 Creating a Calorie Deficit

To lose weight, you need to create a calorie deficit by consuming fewer calories than your body needs. A common guideline is to aim for a deficit of 500 to 1000 calories per day, which can result in a safe and sustainable weight loss of about 1 to 2 pounds per week.

Conclusion

Understanding calories is fundamental to your rapid weight loss journey. By grasping the science of calories and calculating your daily calorie needs, you can make informed dietary decisions that align with your weight loss goals. Keep in mind that while calorie counting is a useful tool, the quality of the calories you consume also plays a crucial role in your overall health and success in achieving and maintaining a healthy weight.

Chapter 7:

Meal Planning and Preparation

Introduction

Effective meal planning and preparation are essential components of a successful rapid weight loss strategy. In Chapter 7, we explore the strategies for weekly meal planning, batch cooking, and provide nutrient-rich and calorie-friendly recipes to help you stay on track.

Section 1: Weekly Meal Planning Strategies

1.1 The Benefits of Meal Planning

Meal planning offers several advantages for weight loss:

1.1.1 Portion Control

By planning meals in advance, you can control portion sizes and avoid overeating.

1.1.2 Nutritional Balance

You can ensure that your meals are balanced, incorporating a variety of macronutrients and micronutrients.

1.1.3 Reduced Food Waste

Planning helps you use ingredients efficiently, reducing food waste.

1.2 Steps for Effective Meal Planning

1.2.1 Set Goals

Determine your daily calorie target and macronutrient goals. This provides a clear framework for your meal planning.

1.2.2 Choose Recipes

Select recipes that align with your goals and preferences. Look for nutrient-rich, lower-calorie options.

1.2.3 Create a Shopping List

Based on your chosen recipes, create a shopping list. Stick to it to minimize impulse purchases.

1.2.4 Prep Ingredients

Wash, chop, and prepare ingredients in advance to streamline meal preparation during the week.

1.2.5 Schedule Meals

Plan your meals for the week, considering your schedule and commitments. Be realistic about what you can cook each day.

Section 2: Batch Cooking and Meal Prep

2.1 The Power of Batch Cooking

Batch cooking involves preparing multiple servings of a dish to be enjoyed throughout the week. It's a time-saving strategy that promotes healthier eating.

2.1.1 Ideal Batch Cooking Dishes

Opt for dishes that reheat well, such as soups, stews, roasted vegetables, and whole grains like quinoa or brown rice.

2.1.2 Portion and Freeze

Divide batch-cooked meals into individual portions and freeze them. This prevents overeating and makes it easy to grab a healthy meal when you're busy.

2.2 Meal Prep Tips

2.2.1 Efficient Tools

Invest in meal prep containers, food scales, and storage solutions to make meal prep seamless.

2.2.2 Plan for Snacks

Prepare healthy snacks like cut-up vegetables, Greek yogurt, or mixed nuts in portioned containers.

2.2.3 Versatile Ingredients

Choose versatile ingredients that can be used in multiple dishes throughout the week. For example, roast a variety of vegetables to add to salads, wraps, and grain bowls.

Section 3: Nutrient-Rich and Calorie-Friendly Recipes

3.1 Breakfast Recipes

3.1.1 Greek Yogurt Parfait

Layer Greek yogurt with fresh berries and a sprinkle of granola for a protein-packed breakfast.

3.1.2 Veggie Omelet

Whisk eggs with diced bell peppers, onions, and spinach for a low-calorie, high-protein breakfast.

3.2 Lunch Recipes

3.2.1 Quinoa Salad

Toss cooked quinoa with diced cucumbers, cherry tomatoes, fresh herbs, and a lemon vinaigrette.

3.2.2 Turkey and Avocado Wrap

Fill whole-grain wraps with lean turkey, avocado slices, lettuce, and a drizzle of mustard.

3.3 Dinner Recipes

3.3.1 Baked Salmon

Season salmon fillets with lemon, garlic, and herbs, then bake for a nutritious dinner.

3.3.2 Vegetable Stir-Fry

Stir-fry a mix of colorful vegetables with tofu or lean chicken, using a low-sodium sauce.

3.4 Snack Ideas

3.4.1 Hummus and Veggies

Dip carrot and cucumber sticks into hummus for a satisfying snack.

3.4.2 Cottage Cheese and Pineapple

Pair low-fat cottage cheese with fresh pineapple chunks.

Conclusion

Meal planning, batch cooking, and the use of nutrient-rich, calorie-friendly recipes are powerful tools in your rapid weight loss journey. By adopting these strategies, you can maintain portion control, achieve nutritional balance, reduce food waste, and save time while enjoying delicious, satisfying meals that support your weight loss goals. Remember that consistency and variety are key to long-term success, so continue exploring new recipes and adapting your meal planning to suit your evolving needs and tastes.

Chapter 8:

Managing Hunger and Cravings

Introduction

Successfully managing hunger and cravings is a critical aspect of any rapid weight loss plan. In Chapter 8, we'll explore the science of satiety and appetite control, provide a list of healthy snack options, and offer strategies to help you handle cravings effectively.

Section 1: Satiety and Appetite Control

1.1 Understanding Satiety

Satiety refers to the feeling of fullness and satisfaction you experience after a meal. It's a complex process influenced by various factors, including the type of foods you eat and your eating habits.

1.1.1 Fiber-Rich Foods

Incorporate foods high in dietary fiber, such as whole grains, legumes, fruits, and vegetables, into your meals. Fiber promotes feelings of fullness and can help control appetite.

1.1.2 Protein

Include lean protein sources like poultry, fish, tofu, and beans in your meals. Protein-rich foods increase satiety and reduce overall calorie intake.

1.1.3 Healthy Fats

Don't shy away from healthy fats like avocados, nuts, and olive oil. These fats contribute to a sense of satisfaction after eating.

1.2 Mindful Eating

Practicing mindful eating techniques can help you tune into your body's hunger and fullness cues.

1.2.1 Slow Down

Eat slowly and savor each bite. It takes time for your body to register fullness.

1.2.2 Portion Control

Use smaller plates and bowls to control portion sizes. This can prevent overeating.

1.2.3 Pay Attention

Eat without distractions, such as television or smartphones. Focus on the sensory experience of eating.

Section 2: Healthy Snack Options

2.1 Nutrient-Rich Snacks

Healthy snacks can keep your energy levels stable between meals and prevent overindulging. Consider these options:

2.1.1 Greek Yogurt

Greek yogurt is high in protein and makes a satisfying snack. Add berries and a drizzle of honey for sweetness.

2.1.2 Mixed Nuts

A small handful of unsalted mixed nuts provides healthy fats and protein to curb cravings.

2.1.3 Vegetable Sticks and Hummus

Carrot, cucumber, and bell pepper sticks paired with hummus make a crunchy and nutritious snack.

2.2 Balanced Snack Combos

Combine macronutrients to create satisfying snacks:

2.2.1 Apple and Almond Butter

Pair apple slices with a tablespoon of almond butter for a sweet and satisfying snack.

2.2.2 Cottage Cheese and Pineapple

Combine low-fat cottage cheese with fresh pineapple chunks for a protein-packed snack.

2.2.3 Hard-Boiled Eggs

Hard-boiled eggs are rich in protein. Sprinkle them with a pinch of salt and pepper for flavor.

Section 3: Strategies for Handling Cravings

3.1 Identify Triggers

Understanding what triggers your cravings can help you manage them more effectively.

3.1.1 Emotional Eating

If stress or emotions drive your cravings, seek alternative ways to cope, such as meditation, exercise, or talking to a friend.

3.1.2 Environmental Triggers

Identify specific environments or situations that lead to cravings and make efforts to avoid or manage them.

3.2 Plan for Indulgences

It's okay to indulge occasionally. Plan for controlled, small treats to satisfy cravings without derailing your progress.

3.2.1 Portion Control

Enjoy your favorite treat in moderation, savoring each bite.

3.2.2 Substitute Smartly

Find healthier alternatives for your favorite indulgences. For example, opt for dark chocolate instead of milk chocolate.

3.3 Stay Hydrated

Dehydration can sometimes be mistaken for hunger. Drink water throughout the day to stay adequately hydrated.

3.4 Distract Yourself

When a craving strikes, engage in a distracting activity to shift your focus away from food. Take a walk, read a book, or work on a hobby.

Conclusion

Effectively managing hunger and cravings is essential for staying on track with your rapid weight loss goals. By understanding satiety, choosing nutrient-rich snacks, and implementing strategies for handling cravings, you can develop a healthier relationship with food and make choices that align with your objectives. Remember that occasional indulgences are normal, and it's the overall consistency and balance in your approach to eating that lead to long-term success.

Chapter 9:

Specialized Diet Plans

Introduction

Specialized diet plans have gained popularity for their potential to aid in rapid weight loss. In Chapter 9, we'll explore several of these plans, including low-carb diets, intermittent fasting, plant-based diets, and others. Understanding the principles and considerations of these diets can help you make informed choices that align with your weight loss goals.

Section 1: Low-Carb Diets

1.1 Understanding Low-Carb Diets

Low-carb diets, such as the Atkins Diet and the Ketogenic Diet (Keto), restrict carbohydrate intake and emphasize higher consumption of proteins and fats. The goal is to shift your body into a state of ketosis, where it primarily burns fat for energy.

1.1.1 Key Principles

- Focus on foods like meat, fish, eggs, nuts, and non-starchy vegetables.

- Limit or eliminate sugary foods, grains, and high-carb fruits.

- Monitor daily carbohydrate intake to stay within your target range.

1.1.2 Considerations

Low-carb diets can be effective for rapid weight loss but may require careful planning to ensure nutrient adequacy. Consult with a healthcare professional before starting.

Section 2: Intermittent Fasting

2.1 Understanding Intermittent Fasting

Intermittent fasting involves cycling between periods of eating and fasting. Common approaches include the 16/8 method (16 hours of fasting with an 8-hour eating window) and the 5:2 method (eating normally for 5 days and restricting calorie intake on 2 non-consecutive days).

2.1.1 Benefits

- Potential for weight loss due to reduced calorie intake.

- Possible improvements in insulin sensitivity and cellular repair.

2.1.2 Considerations

Intermittent fasting may not be suitable for everyone. Consult with a healthcare provider, especially if you have underlying health conditions.

Section 3: Plant-Based Diets

3.1 Understanding Plant-Based Diets

Plant-based diets emphasize foods derived from plants, including fruits, vegetables, legumes, nuts, and seeds. While plant-based diets vary (from vegetarian to vegan), they often focus on whole, unprocessed foods.

3.1.1 Benefits

- Potential for weight loss due to the high fiber content and lower calorie density of plant-based foods.

- Health benefits, including reduced risk of chronic diseases.

3.1.2 Considerations

Ensure proper nutrient intake, especially for protein, vitamin B12, and iron, when following a plant-based diet. Consult a healthcare provider or dietitian for guidance.

Section 4: Other Specialized Diets

4.1 Keto Diet

4.1.1 Key Principles

The Keto Diet is a high-fat, low-carb diet designed to induce ketosis. It involves a strict restriction of carbohydrates and emphasizes fats and moderate protein.

4.1.2 Considerations

Keto can be effective for weight loss, but it may be challenging to sustain long-term. It requires careful planning and monitoring.

4.2 Paleo Diet

4.2.1 Key Principles

The Paleo Diet focuses on foods presumed to have been available to early humans, such as lean meats, fish, fruits, vegetables, nuts, and seeds. It excludes processed foods, dairy, grains, and legumes.

4.2.2 Considerations

While the Paleo Diet can promote weight loss, it may be restrictive and may not provide all essential nutrients. Consult a healthcare provider.

4.3 Mediterranean Diet

4.3.1 Key Principles

The Mediterranean Diet emphasizes fruits, vegetables, whole grains, fish, and healthy fats like olive oil. It's associated with heart health and may support weight loss.

4.3.2 Considerations

The Mediterranean Diet is generally considered a balanced and sustainable approach to weight management and overall health.

Conclusion

Specialized diet plans offer various approaches to rapid weight loss. Each has its own principles, benefits, and considerations. Before embarking on any specialized diet, consult with a healthcare provider or registered dietitian to ensure it's appropriate for your individual needs and to receive personalized guidance. Remember that long-term success depends on finding a sustainable dietary approach that aligns with your lifestyle and preferences.

Chapter 10:

Hydration and Supplements

Hydration and dietary supplements can play a role in supporting your rapid weight loss journey. Chapter 10 delves into the significance of water consumption, explores supplements that may aid in weight loss, and highlights potential pitfalls associated with supplementation.

Section 1: The Importance of Water

1.1 The Role of Hydration

Proper hydration is crucial for overall health and can have a significant impact on your weight loss efforts.

1.1.1 Appetite Control

Drinking water before meals can help control appetite and reduce calorie intake.

1.1.2 Metabolism Support

Adequate hydration supports metabolic processes, including the breakdown of stored fat for energy.

1.1.3 Energy Levels

Staying hydrated helps maintain energy levels, making it easier to engage in physical activity.

1.2 Tips for Staying Hydrated

1.2.1 Water Consumption

Aim for at least eight 8-ounce glasses of water per day, but individual needs may vary.

1.2.2 Listen to Your Body

Pay attention to thirst cues and drink water when you're thirsty.

1.2.3 Hydrating Foods

Incorporate water-rich foods like fruits and vegetables into your diet.

Section 2: Supplements That May Aid Weight Loss

2.1 Weight Loss Supplements

Several dietary supplements are marketed as weight loss aids. Some of the most commonly mentioned include:

2.1.1 Green Tea Extract

Green tea extract contains compounds like catechins that may boost metabolism and aid in fat burning.

2.1.2 Garcinia Cambogia

Garcinia cambogia is believed to suppress appetite and inhibit fat storage.

2.1.3 Caffeine

Caffeine is a natural stimulant that can temporarily increase metabolic rate and energy expenditure.

2.2 Considerations for Supplements

2.2.1 Research and Safety

Before taking any supplement, research its safety and efficacy. Consult with a healthcare provider to ensure it won't interact with medications or have adverse effects.

2.2.2 No Magic Pill

Supplements are not a substitute for a healthy diet and exercise. Their effects are often modest, and they work best when combined with a balanced lifestyle.

Section 3: Potential Pitfalls of Supplementation

3.1 Unregulated Market

The dietary supplement industry is largely unregulated, which can lead to issues such as:

3.1.1 Lack of Efficacy

Some supplements may not contain the ingredients or concentrations they claim.

3.1.2 Contamination

Contaminated supplements may pose health risks.

3.2 Side Effects

Supplements, even natural ones, can have side effects and may not be suitable for everyone.

3.2.1 Gastrointestinal Issues

Some supplements can cause digestive discomfort.

3.2.2 Cardiovascular Effects

Stimulant-based supplements can affect heart rate and blood pressure.

3.3 Financial Costs

Supplements can be expensive, and the cost can add up over time.

3.4 Psychological Dependency

Relying on supplements for weight loss may not address the underlying behaviors and habits contributing to weight gain.

Conclusion

Hydration and supplements can be tools in your rapid weight loss journey, but they should be used judiciously and with caution. Prioritize proper hydration, as it supports overall health and can aid in weight loss. When considering supplements, research their safety and efficacy, and consult with a healthcare provider. Remember that there is no magic pill for weight loss, and long-term success depends on a balanced and sustainable approach that includes a healthy diet, regular physical activity, and a focus on overall well-being.

Part 3:
Exercise and Physical Activity

Chapter 11:

Crafting Your Workout Plan

Introduction

Exercise is a fundamental component of any effective weight loss strategy. Chapter 11 is dedicated to helping you craft a personalized workout plan that aligns with your rapid weight loss goals. We'll explore different types of exercises, including cardiovascular, strength training, and flexibility workouts, and provide guidance on finding the right routine for you.

Section 1: Cardiovascular Exercises

1.1 The Role of Cardiovascular Exercises

Cardiovascular exercises, often referred to as *"cardio,"* are activities that elevate your heart rate and increase oxygen consumption. They play a crucial role in burning calories and improving cardiovascular health.

1.1.1 Benefits

- **Calorie Burn:** Cardio exercises help create a calorie deficit, promoting weight loss.

- **Improved Heart Health:** Regular cardio can enhance cardiovascular fitness and reduce the risk of heart disease.

- **Stress Reduction:** Cardio workouts release endorphins, reducing stress and improving mood.

1.2 Types of Cardio Exercises

1.2.1 Running and Jogging

1.2.2 Cycling

1.2.3 Swimming

1.2.4 Jump Rope

1.2.5 Aerobic Classes

Section 2: Strength Training

2.1 The Importance of Strength Training

Strength training involves resistance exercises that build muscle mass and boost metabolism. It's a valuable addition to your workout plan for weight loss.

2.1.1 Benefits

- **Increased Muscle Mass:** More muscle means a higher resting metabolic rate.

- **Calorie Burn:** Strength training burns calories during and after workouts.

- **Improved Body Composition:** Builds lean muscle and reduces body fat.

2.2 Types of Strength Training

2.2.1 Free Weights

2.2.2 Resistance Bands

2.2.3 Bodyweight Exercises

2.2.4 Machines

Section 3: Flexibility and Mobility Workouts

3.1 The Role of Flexibility and Mobility

Flexibility and mobility workouts enhance joint range of motion, reduce the risk of injury, and improve overall physical function.

3.1.1 Benefits

- **Injury Prevention:** Enhanced flexibility reduces the risk of strains and sprains.

- **Posture and Alignment:** Better mobility supports proper posture and alignment.

- **Stress Reduction:** These workouts can promote relaxation and stress relief.

3.2 Types of Flexibility and Mobility Workouts

3.2.1 Yoga

3.2.2 Pilates

3.2.3 Stretching Routines

3.2.4 Foam Rolling

Section 4: Finding the Right Workout Routine for You

4.1 Individual Preferences

Consider your personal preferences when crafting your workout plan. What types of exercises do you enjoy? Incorporating activities you like can make it more likely that you'll stick to your routine.

4.2 Fitness Level

Assess your current fitness level and tailor your workouts accordingly. Gradually progress to more challenging exercises as your strength and stamina improve.

4.3 Time Commitment

Determine how much time you can realistically dedicate to exercise. Even short, intense workouts can be effective for weight loss.

4.4 Variety

Incorporate variety into your routine to prevent boredom and reduce the risk of overuse injuries. Alternate between cardio, strength training, and flexibility workouts.

4.5 Professional Guidance

Consider seeking guidance from a certified fitness trainer or coach. They can help you create a customized workout plan and ensure proper form and technique.

Conclusion

Crafting a personalized workout plan that includes cardiovascular exercises, strength training, and flexibility workouts is a key component of your rapid weight loss journey. Remember that consistency and gradual progression are essential for long-term success. Choose activities you enjoy, listen to your body, and adapt your routine as needed. With the right plan in place, you can

achieve your weight loss goals and experience the
many health benefits of regular physical activity.

Chapter 12:

Incorporating Exercise into Your Daily Life

Introduction

While crafting a workout plan is essential, it's equally important to incorporate exercise seamlessly into your daily life. In Chapter 12, we'll explore strategies for building a consistent exercise habit, finding time for workouts, and the pros and cons of home versus gym workouts.

Section 1: Building a Consistent Exercise Habit

1.1 The Power of Habit

Establishing a consistent exercise habit is crucial for long-term success. Habits require less conscious effort and become part of your daily routine.

1.1.1 Start Small

Begin with manageable goals and gradually increase the intensity and duration of your workouts as your habit solidifies.

1.1.2 Set a Schedule

Designate specific days and times for exercise, treating it as an appointment you can't miss.

1.1.3 Accountability

Enlist a workout buddy, join a fitness class, or use fitness apps to help you stay accountable to your routine.

1.2 Mindset Shift

Embrace exercise as a way to enhance your well-being, boost your energy, and reduce stress, rather than solely as a means for weight loss.

Section 2: Finding Time for Workouts

2.1 Prioritizing Exercise

Finding time for workouts requires prioritization and efficient time management.

2.1.1 Time Blocking

Allocate specific time blocks for exercise in your daily or weekly schedule.

2.1.2 Morning Workouts

Morning exercise can jumpstart your day and ensure it doesn't get pushed aside by other commitments.

2.1.3 Short, Intense Workouts

Consider high-intensity interval training (HIIT) or other time-efficient workouts that deliver results in a shorter time frame.

Section 3: Home vs. Gym Workouts

3.1 Home Workouts

3.1.1 Pros

- Convenience: No commute to the gym.

- Cost-Effective: No membership fees.

- Privacy: Workout at your own pace.

3.1.2 Cons

- Limited Equipment: May require investing in home gym equipment.

- Distractions: Potential distractions at home.

- Social Interaction: May miss the social aspect of a gym.

3.2 Gym Workouts

3.2.1 Pros

- Equipment Variety: Access to a wide range of exercise equipment.

- Motivation: Gym atmosphere can be motivating.

- Social Interaction: Opportunity to meet others with similar fitness goals.

3.2.2 Cons

- Time-Consuming: Traveling to and from the gym can be time-consuming.

- Cost: Gym memberships often come with a monthly fee.

- Crowds: Peak gym hours can be crowded.

Conclusion

Incorporating exercise into your daily life is essential for achieving and maintaining rapid weight loss. Building a consistent exercise habit, finding time for workouts, and choosing between home and gym workouts are all important considerations. The key is to find an approach that aligns with your lifestyle, preferences, and goals. Regardless of where or how you exercise, the most crucial factor is staying committed and making physical activity an integral part of your daily routine.

Chapter 13:

Tracking Progress

Introduction

Monitoring your fitness and weight loss progress is crucial for staying on course and making informed adjustments to your rapid weight loss journey. In Chapter 13, we'll explore the importance of tracking your progress, methods for measuring body composition changes, and the benefits of using fitness apps and wearables.

Section 1: Monitoring Fitness and Weight Loss Progress

1.1 Why Track Progress

Tracking your progress provides several key benefits:

1.1.1 Motivation

Seeing tangible progress can boost your motivation and reinforce your commitment to your goals.

1.1.2 Accountability

Regular tracking holds you accountable for your actions and keeps you mindful of your efforts.

1.1.3 Course Correction

By monitoring your progress, you can identify areas where you need to make adjustments to your diet or exercise routine.

1.2 Methods of Tracking

1.2.1 Weighing Scale

Regular weigh-ins can provide insights into changes in body weight, although it's important to remember that weight fluctuations are normal.

1.2.2 Body Measurements

Measuring key areas of your body, such as waist, hips, and thighs, can help you track changes in body composition.

1.2.3 Progress Photos

Taking photos at regular intervals can visually document your transformation and reveal changes that might not be apparent on the scale.

Section 2: Measuring Body Composition Changes

2.1 Beyond the Scale

While weight is a valuable metric, it doesn't tell the whole story. Measuring body composition provides a more accurate picture of your progress.

2.1.1 Body Fat Percentage

Body fat percentage is a critical indicator of progress. Methods for measuring body fat include skinfold calipers, bioelectrical impedance scales, and DEXA scans.

2.1.2 Lean Body Mass

Tracking lean body mass (muscle mass) helps ensure that weight loss is primarily from fat, not muscle.

2.2 Professional Assessments

Consider consulting with a fitness professional or registered dietitian for a comprehensive assessment of your body composition and progress.

Section 3: Using Fitness Apps and Wearables

3.1 The Role of Technology

Fitness apps and wearables have revolutionized the way we track progress by making it more convenient and accessible.

3.1.1 Tracking Workouts

Fitness apps can log your workouts, monitor your heart rate, and estimate calorie burn.

3.1.2 Dietary Tracking

Apps can help you log your food intake, providing insights into your nutritional habits.

3.1.3 Setting Goals

Many apps allow you to set and track specific fitness and weight loss goals.

3.2 Choosing the Right Tools

Select fitness apps and wearables that align with your goals and preferences. Look for features that support your specific needs, whether it's tracking running, cycling, strength training, or overall health and wellness.

Conclusion

Tracking your fitness and weight loss progress is a valuable tool for achieving your rapid weight loss goals. It offers motivation, accountability, and the ability to make informed adjustments to your plan. Whether you prefer traditional methods like the scale and tape measure or opt for modern technology with fitness apps and wearables, the important thing is to remain consistent in your tracking efforts. By doing so, you'll have a clearer understanding of your progress and be better equipped to stay on the path to success.

Chapter 14:

Overcoming Exercise Plateaus

Introduction

Exercise plateaus are common during a weight loss journey. In Chapter 14, we'll explore strategies for dealing with workout plateaus, the importance of varying your exercise routine, and the role of rest and recovery in breaking through stagnation.

Section 1: Dealing with Workout Plateaus

1.1 Recognizing Plateaus

Plateaus occur when your progress slows down or comes to a halt, despite consistent effort. They can be frustrating, but they are a natural part of the fitness journey.

1.1.1 Common Signs

- No change in weight or body measurements.

- Decreased performance during workouts.

- A lack of motivation or enthusiasm.

1.2 Strategies for Overcoming Plateaus

1.2.1 Progressive Overload

Gradually increase the intensity, duration, or resistance in your workouts to challenge your body and stimulate further progress.

1.2.2 Change Exercise Variables

Alter exercise selection, order, and intensity to surprise your muscles and break the monotony.

1.2.3 Mix Cardio and Strength

Combine cardiovascular workouts with strength training to engage different muscle groups and energy systems.

Section 2: Varying Your Exercise Routine

2.1 Importance of Variety

Varying your exercise routine not only prevents plateaus but also keeps your workouts engaging and enjoyable.

2.1.1 Muscle Confusion

Changing exercises regularly can prevent your muscles from adapting to a specific routine.

2.1.2 Mental Stimulation

New exercises or activities can challenge you mentally, keeping your workouts fresh and interesting.

2.2 Exploring Different Workouts

2.2.1 Cross-Training

Incorporate activities like swimming, cycling, or yoga to add variety and reduce the risk of overuse injuries.

2.2.2 Group Classes

Join fitness classes or group activities to add a social element and expose yourself to different workout styles.

2.2.3 Outdoor Workouts

Take advantage of outdoor activities like hiking, trail running, or outdoor circuit training to change your workout environment.

Section 3: The Role of Rest and Recovery

3.1 Importance of Rest

Rest and recovery are essential components of any exercise program. They allow your body to repair and adapt.

3.1.1 Muscle Repair

Rest allows muscles to recover, repair, and grow stronger.

3.1.2 Injury Prevention

Adequate rest helps prevent overuse injuries and burnout.

3.2 Structured Rest

3.2.1 Rest Days

Incorporate regular rest days into your workout schedule to allow your body to fully recover.

3.2.2 Deload Weeks

Periodically reduce workout intensity and volume to give your body a break and prevent overtraining.

3.2.3 Sleep

Prioritize quality sleep to support recovery and overall well-being.

Conclusion

Dealing with workout plateaus is a normal part of any fitness journey, but with the right strategies, you can overcome them and continue progressing toward your weight loss goals. Remember the importance of progressive overload, varying your exercise routine, and allowing your body sufficient rest and recovery. By embracing change, challenging yourself, and taking care of your body, you can push through plateaus and experience continued growth and success in your fitness journey.

Part 4:

Mindset and Lifestyle

Chapter 15:

Managing Stress and Sleep

Introduction

Stress management and quality sleep play significant roles in your overall well-being and can impact your weight loss journey. Chapter 15 focuses on understanding the impact of stress on weight loss, strategies for managing stress, and the importance of prioritizing quality sleep.

Section 1: Stress's Impact on Weight Loss

1.1 The Stress-Weight Connection

Chronic stress can affect your weight loss efforts in several ways:

1.1.1 Hormonal Changes

Stress triggers the release of cortisol, a hormone that can lead to increased fat storage, particularly in the abdominal area.

1.1.2 Emotional Eating

Stress can lead to emotional eating, where you turn to food for comfort or as a coping mechanism.

1.2 Recognizing Stress Eating

1.2.1 Mindful Eating

Practicing mindful eating can help you become aware of emotional eating triggers and develop healthier responses.

1.2.2 Stress-Reduction Techniques

Incorporate stress-reduction techniques, such as meditation, deep breathing, or yoga, into your daily routine to mitigate emotional eating.

Section 2: Strategies for Stress Management

2.1 Stress Reduction Techniques

2.1.1 Exercise

Regular physical activity is a powerful stress reducer, releasing endorphins that improve mood and reduce stress.

2.1.2 Mindfulness and Meditation

Mindfulness practices and meditation can help you manage stress by increasing self-awareness and promoting relaxation.

2.2 Time Management

Effective time management can reduce stress by allowing you to allocate time for self-care, exercise, and relaxation.

2.2.1 Prioritization

Identify your priorities and allocate time accordingly to reduce the feeling of being overwhelmed.

2.2.2 Boundaries

Set boundaries to prevent overcommitting and create space for self-care activities.

Section 3: The Importance of Quality Sleep

3.1 Sleep and Weight Loss

Quality sleep is essential for weight loss and overall health:

3.1.1 Hormonal Balance

Sleep regulates hormones like leptin and ghrelin, which control appetite and hunger.

3.1.2 Energy Levels

Adequate sleep improves energy levels and supports physical activity.

3.2 Sleep Hygiene

3.2.1 Consistent Schedule

Maintain a regular sleep schedule by going to bed and waking up at the same time each day.

3.2.2 Sleep Environment

Create a sleep-conducive environment with a comfortable mattress, proper room temperature, and minimal light and noise.

3.2.3 Bedtime Routine

Establish a relaxing bedtime routine to signal to your body that it's time to wind down.

Conclusion

Managing stress and prioritizing quality sleep are vital components of your weight loss journey and overall well-being. Recognize the impact of stress on weight loss, adopt stress-reduction strategies, and prioritize self-care. Equally important is ensuring you get adequate, restorative sleep to support your physical and emotional health. By managing stress and optimizing your sleep habits, you'll create a more favorable environment for successful weight loss and a healthier lifestyle.

Chapter 16:

Maintaining Motivation

Introduction

Maintaining motivation throughout your weight loss journey is essential for long-term success. In Chapter 16, we'll explore strategies for staying motivated, including setting mini-goals, visualizing success, and using positive reinforcement and rewards.

Section 1: Setting Mini-Goals

1.1 The Power of Mini-Goals

Breaking your weight loss journey into smaller, achievable goals can provide a sense of accomplishment and help you stay motivated.

1.1.1 Specific Goals

Set clear and specific mini-goals, such as losing a certain amount of weight, running a certain distance, or fitting into a specific clothing size.

1.1.2 Measurable Progress

Track your progress toward each mini-goal to see your achievements over time.

1.2 Celebrating Milestones

1.2.1 Rewards

Celebrate reaching mini-goals with rewards that are not food-related, such as treating yourself to a new workout outfit or a relaxing spa day.

1.2.2 Reflection

Take time to reflect on your achievements and acknowledge your dedication and hard work.

Section 2: Visualizing Success

2.1 The Power of Visualization

Visualizing your success can help you stay motivated by creating a mental image of your desired outcomes.

2.1.1 Create a Vision Board

Compile images, quotes, and reminders of your goals and place them on a vision board you can see regularly.

2.1.2 Mental Rehearsal

Mentally rehearse your success by imagining yourself reaching your goals and experiencing the positive emotions that come with it.

2.2 Positive Self-Talk

Use positive affirmations and self-talk to reinforce your belief in your ability to achieve your weight loss goals.

2.2.1 Challenge Negative Thoughts

Challenge and replace negative self-talk with positive and empowering statements.

2.2.2 Encourage Yourself

Be your own cheerleader, offering words of encouragement and support during challenging times.

Section 3: Positive Reinforcement and Rewards

3.1 The Role of Rewards

Using positive reinforcement and rewards can help reinforce good habits and maintain motivation.

3.1.1 Intrinsic Rewards

Find joy and satisfaction in the process itself, such as the sense of accomplishment from completing a challenging workout.

3.1.2 Extrinsic Rewards

Occasionally treat yourself with rewards like a favorite book, a movie night, or a special outing for achieving significant milestones.

3.2 Tracking Progress

Keep a record of your achievements and use it as a reminder of how far you've come.

3.2.1 Progress Journal

Maintain a journal to record your weight loss journey, including successes, setbacks, and lessons learned.

3.2.2 Visual Tracking

Create visual trackers, such as a chart or graph, to visualize your progress and see the positive trends.

Conclusion

Maintaining motivation is a key factor in the success of your weight loss journey. By setting mini-goals, visualizing success, and using positive reinforcement and rewards, you can stay focused and inspired along the way. Remember that motivation may ebb and flow, but with these strategies in place, you'll have the tools to reignite your enthusiasm and continue making progress toward your weight loss goals.

Chapter 17:

Handling Setbacks and Challenges

Introduction

Setbacks and challenges are inevitable on your weight loss journey. Chapter 17 is dedicated to equipping you with strategies for dealing with obstacles, avoiding common pitfalls, and effectively bouncing back from indulgences.

Section 1: Strategies for Dealing with Obstacles

1.1 Identifying Common Obstacles

Recognizing the challenges you might face on your weight loss journey is the first step in overcoming them.

1.1.1 Emotional Eating

Learn to distinguish between emotional hunger and physical hunger to avoid turning to food as a coping mechanism.

1.1.2 Plateaus

Understand that weight loss plateaus are normal and can often be overcome with adjustments to your diet or exercise routine.

1.2 Problem-Solving

1.2.1 Setting Realistic Expectations

Ensure your goals are achievable and realistic to prevent discouragement.

1.2.2 Seeking Support

Don't hesitate to reach out to friends, family, or a support group when facing challenges. Talking through your obstacles can provide valuable insights and encouragement.

Section 2: Avoiding Common Pitfalls

2.1 Common Weight Loss Pitfalls

Awareness of common pitfalls can help you steer clear of them.

2.1.1 All-or-Nothing Thinking

Avoid the trap of thinking that one slip-up ruins your progress. Perfection is not required; consistency is key.

2.1.2 Over-Restricting

Excessive calorie restriction or overly strict diets are difficult to maintain long-term and can lead to binge eating.

2.2 Sustainable Habits

2.2.1 Focus on Habits

Shift your focus from quick fixes to building sustainable, healthy habits that you can maintain over time.

2.2.2 Mindful Eating

Practice mindful eating to enhance your awareness of hunger cues, satiety, and food choices.

Section 3: Bouncing Back from Indulgences

3.1 Treating Indulgences Mindfully

Occasional indulgences are part of a balanced lifestyle. Instead of guilt, approach them with mindfulness.

3.1.1 Enjoy Without Guilt

Allow yourself to savor indulgent foods without feeling guilty. Savoring can reduce the urge to overindulge.

3.1.2 Balance and Moderation

Balance indulgences with healthier choices before and after to maintain your overall dietary balance.

3.2 Rebounding After Indulgences

3.2.1 Get Back on Track

After an indulgence, resume your regular eating and exercise routine without delay.

3.2.2 Self-Compassion

Practice self-compassion and avoid self-criticism. One indulgence does not define your entire journey.

Conclusion

Setbacks and challenges are a natural part of any weight loss journey. By recognizing and strategizing for obstacles, avoiding common pitfalls, and approaching indulgences mindfully, you can overcome setbacks and continue progressing toward your goals. Remember that setbacks do not define your journey; your ability to adapt and persevere in the face of challenges is a true testament to your dedication and determination.

Chapter 18:

Long-Term Weight Maintenance

Introduction

Long-term weight maintenance is the ultimate goal of any successful weight loss journey. Chapter 18 focuses on transitioning to a lifelong healthy lifestyle, providing strategies for maintaining weight loss, and celebrating and reflecting on your journey.

Section 1: Transitioning to a Lifelong Healthy Lifestyle

1.1 Shifting Perspective

Transitioning from a weight loss mindset to a lifelong healthy lifestyle perspective is essential for lasting success.

1.1.1 Sustainable Habits

Continue practicing the healthy habits you developed during your weight loss journey, making them a permanent part of your lifestyle.

1.1.2 Enjoyment

Find joy in healthy eating and regular physical activity to ensure long-term commitment.

1.2 Mindful Eating

1.2.1 Intuitive Eating

Embrace intuitive eating, focusing on internal hunger and satiety cues rather than external rules.

1.2.2 Flexibility

Allow flexibility in your eating habits, understanding that occasional indulgences are part of a balanced life.

Section 2: Strategies for Maintaining Weight Loss

2.1 Continued Tracking

Maintaining awareness of your progress and habits is crucial for weight maintenance.

2.1.1 Regular Weigh-Ins

Continue weighing yourself regularly to catch any potential weight gain early.

2.1.2 Food Journaling

Keep a food journal to monitor your eating habits and identify areas where adjustments may be needed.

2.2 Staying Active

2.2.1 Consistent Exercise

Maintain a consistent exercise routine that includes a combination of cardiovascular, strength training, and flexibility exercises.

2.2.2 Daily Activity

Incorporate physical activity into your daily life, such as walking, taking the stairs, or engaging in active hobbies.

Section 3: Celebrating and Reflecting on Your Journey

3.1 Celebrating Success

Celebrate your achievements and milestones to stay motivated and reinforce your commitment to a healthy lifestyle.

3.1.1 Non-Food Rewards

Reward yourself with non-food items or experiences when you achieve significant goals.

3.1.2 Gratitude

Practice gratitude for the positive changes you've made and the benefits of a healthier lifestyle.

3.2 Reflecting on the Journey

Take time to reflect on your weight loss journey and the lessons you've learned along the way.

3.2.1 Journaling

Maintain a journal to document your experiences, challenges, and successes.

3.2.2 Sharing Your Story

Consider sharing your journey with others to inspire and support those on a similar path.

Conclusion

Long-term weight maintenance is the culmination of your efforts and dedication to a healthier lifestyle. By shifting your perspective, practicing mindful eating, and staying active, you can ensure lasting success. Celebrate your achievements and reflect on your journey to reinforce your commitment and inspire others. Remember that maintaining a healthy weight is not just about the destination but about the journey itself—a journey toward improved well-being and a higher quality of life.

Conclusion

Congratulations on completing your 30-day transformation journey towards a healthier lifestyle! Over the past month, you've embarked on a remarkable and impactful journey, making positive changes in various aspects of your life. Let's take a moment to reflect on your achievements and look forward to continuing your journey towards a healthy and fulfilling lifestyle.

Reflecting on Your 30-Day Transformation

During this transformative period, you've:

- **Focused on Nutrition:** You've learned about the science of weight loss, understood the importance of calorie management, and explored meal planning and preparation to fuel your body with nutritious foods.

- **Prioritized Physical Activity:** You've crafted a personalized workout plan, incorporating cardiovascular exercises, strength training, and flexibility workouts to enhance your fitness.

- **Embraced a Healthier Mindset:** You've discovered strategies for maintaining motivation, handling setbacks, and transitioning to a lifelong healthy lifestyle.

- **Monitored Progress:** You've learned how to track your fitness and weight loss journey, measure body composition changes, and leverage technology with fitness apps and wearables.

- **Managed Stress and Sleep:** You've understood the impact of stress on weight loss, adopted stress management techniques, and recognized the importance of quality sleep in your overall well-being.

- **Prepared for Long-Term Success:** You've explored strategies for maintaining weight loss, handling setbacks, and celebrating your journey's achievements.

Encouragement to Continue a Healthy Lifestyle

Your 30-day transformation is just the beginning. The habits and knowledge you've gained during this period are invaluable assets as you move forward. Here's some encouragement to keep you motivated:

1. **Consistency Is Key:** Continue practicing the healthy habits you've developed. Consistency over time is the foundation of lasting change.

2. **Be Kind to Yourself:** Remember that setbacks and challenges are part of the journey. Approach them with resilience and a positive attitude.

3. **Set New Goals:** Consider setting new health and wellness goals to keep your journey exciting and inspiring.

4. **Seek Support:** Lean on friends, family, or support communities for encouragement and motivation when needed.

5. **Celebrate Every Milestone:** Continue celebrating your successes, both big and small. Recognize your achievements and use them as motivation to reach new heights.

6. **Prioritize Self-Care:** Don't forget the importance of self-care, including stress management and quality sleep, in maintaining your well-being.

7. **Share Your Story:** If you're comfortable, share your journey with others. Your experiences can inspire and support those striving for a healthier lifestyle.

Remember, the path to a healthy lifestyle is a lifelong journey filled with ups and downs. Embrace each day as an opportunity to make choices that align with your well-being and long-term happiness. You've already proven your dedication to a healthier you, and the possibilities for continued growth and success are limitless. Keep moving forward, and may your journey be filled with health, happiness, and fulfillment.

Appendix

Websites:

1. [MyFitnessPal](https://www.myfitnesspal.com/): A popular app and website for tracking calories and exercise, with a large database of foods.

2. [SparkPeople](https://www.sparkpeople.com/): Offers a variety of tools for tracking nutrition, fitness, and goals, along with a supportive community.

3. [Mayo Clinic - Weight Loss](https://www.mayoclinic.org/healthy-lifestyle/nutrition-and-healthy-eating/expert-answers/weight-loss/faq-20427987): Provides evidence-based information and tips for healthy weight loss.

4. [Choose MyPlate](https://www.myplate.gov/): Offers resources and tools for building a healthy plate and making nutritious food choices.

Apps:

1. [MyFitnessPal](https://www.myfitnesspal.com/): Available for iOS and Android, this app helps you track calories, exercise, and nutrition.

2. [Fitbit](https://www.fitbit.com/): Compatible with Fitbit devices, this app tracks activity, sleep, and nutrition.

3. [Cronometer](https://cronometer.com/): A comprehensive nutrition tracker that focuses on micronutrients and is available for iOS and Android.

4. [Lose It!](https://www.loseit.com/): A user-friendly app for tracking food intake, exercise, and weight loss goals, available for iOS and Android.

Further Reading:

1. *"The Obesity Code" by Dr. Jason Fung:* Explores the science of obesity and offers insights into effective weight management strategies.

2. *"Mindless Eating: Why We Eat More Than We Think" by Brian Wansink:* Examines the psychology of eating and provides practical tips for mindful eating.

3. *"Atomic Habits" by James Clear:* Discusses the power of small habits and how they can lead to significant changes in behavior and lifestyle.

4. *"The Power of Now" by Eckhart Tolle:* Offers insights into mindfulness and being present in the

moment, which can be beneficial for stress management and mindful eating.

5. *"The Whole30: The 30-Day Guide to Total Health and Food Freedom" by Melissa Hartwig Urban and Dallas Hartwig:* Provides a structured 30-day program for improving eating habits and overall health.

These additional resources can provide valuable information, tools, and support as you continue your journey toward a healthier lifestyle. Remember that knowledge and ongoing learning are essential components of long-term success.

Sample Meal Plans and Workout Routines

Sample Meal Plans

Meal Plan 1: Balanced Diet

Breakfast:

- Scrambled eggs with spinach and tomatoes

- Whole-grain toast

- A piece of fruit (e.g., an apple or banana)

Lunch:

- Grilled chicken breast salad with mixed greens, cucumbers, and vinaigrette dressing

- Quinoa or brown rice

Snack:

- Greek yogurt with berries and a drizzle of honey

Dinner:

- Baked salmon with lemon and herbs

- Steamed broccoli and carrots

- Mashed sweet potatoes

Snack (if needed):

- Mixed nuts or a small serving of cottage cheese

Meal Plan 2: Low-Carb

Breakfast:

- Vegetable omelette with mushrooms, bell peppers, and cheese

- Avocado slices

Lunch:

- Grilled shrimp or tofu salad with mixed greens, cherry tomatoes, and olive oil dressing

Snack:

- Sliced cucumber and cherry tomatoes with hummus

Dinner:

- Baked chicken thighs with garlic and rosemary

- Roasted Brussels sprouts with olive oil

- Cauliflower rice

Snack (if needed):

- A small serving of full-fat Greek yogurt

Sample Workout Routines

Workout Routine 1: Cardio and Strength

Day 1 - Cardio:

- 30 minutes of brisk walking or jogging

Day 2 - Strength:

- Push-ups (3 sets of 10 reps)

- Bodyweight squats (3 sets of 12 reps)

- Planks (3 sets of 30 seconds)

Day 3 - Rest or Light Activity

Day 4 - Cardio:

- 20 minutes of cycling or swimming

Day 5 - Strength:

- Dumbbell bench press (3 sets of 10 reps)

- Lunges (3 sets of 12 reps per leg)

- Russian twists (3 sets of 15 reps each side)

Day 6 - Rest or Light Activity

Day 7 - Cardio:

- 30 minutes of your choice (running, dancing, or cycling)

Workout Routine 2: Full-Body HIIT (High-Intensity Interval Training)

Day 1 - HIIT:

- Jumping jacks (30 seconds)

- Push-ups (30 seconds)

- Squat jumps (30 seconds)

- Planks (30 seconds)

- Rest (30 seconds)

- Repeat for a total of 3 rounds

Day 2 - Rest or Light Activity

Day 3 - HIIT:

- Burpees (30 seconds)

- Mountain climbers (30 seconds)

- Dumbbell rows (30 seconds)

- Bicycle crunches (30 seconds)

- Rest (30 seconds)

- Repeat for a total of 3 rounds

Day 4 - Rest or Light Activity

Day 5 - HIIT:

- High knees (30 seconds)

- Tricep dips (30 seconds)

- Lateral lunges (30 seconds)

- Russian twists (30 seconds)

- Rest (30 seconds)

- Repeat for a total of 3 rounds

Day 6 - Rest or Light Activity

Day 7 - Cardio or Rest:

- 30 minutes of steady-state cardio (running, cycling, or swimming) or take a full day of rest

These sample meal plans and workout routines can serve as a starting point for your journey to a healthier lifestyle. Remember to tailor them to your individual preferences and needs. It's crucial to consult with a healthcare professional or fitness expert before beginning any new diet or exercise program, especially if you have specific health concerns or conditions.

Success stories and testimonials.

Success stories and testimonials from individuals who have undergone transformations and achieved their health and fitness goals can be incredibly inspiring and motivating. Here are a few excerpts from people who have successfully embraced healthier lifestyles:

Testimonial 1: Jane's Weight Loss Journey

"Before starting my weight loss journey, I felt tired all the time and lacked confidence. I knew it was time for a change. Over the past year, I've lost 40 pounds by making gradual changes to my diet and incorporating regular exercise. Not only do I have more energy, but my self-esteem has soared. I now believe that anything is possible with dedication and the right support."

Testimonial 2: Mike's Fitness Transformation

"As someone who used to struggle with consistency, I decided to commit to a healthier lifestyle. I started with small steps, like daily walks and reducing sugary drinks. Over time, I built up to running, strength training, and a balanced diet. Today, I'm in the best shape of my life, and I've even completed a marathon! It's amazing what you can achieve when you stay committed."

Testimonial 3: Sarah's Journey to Mindful Eating

"I used to have a complicated relationship with food, often turning to emotional eating. Learning about mindful eating was a game-changer for me. It helped me tune into my body's hunger cues and make healthier choices. I've lost 25 pounds and, more importantly, found peace with food. It's not just about the weight; it's about feeling in control and nourishing my body."

Testimonial 4: John's Stress Management Success

"Stress used to be a constant presence in my life, and it took a toll on my health. I began practicing mindfulness meditation and prioritizing self-care. Over time, my stress levels decreased, and I noticed positive changes in my sleep, mood, and overall well-being. Stress no longer controls me; I control it."

These testimonials highlight the power of determination, consistency, and healthy habits in achieving personal goals. Every journey is unique, and while there may be challenges along the way, these success stories show that with the right mindset and support, positive transformations are possible. You too can embark on your own journey to improved health and well-being.